Transform Your Body

The ultimate guide to sustainable weight loss

By

William K. Hawkins

Table of Content

Introduction 4

Understanding the Weight Loss Journey 4

   Setting Realistic Goals 8

Chapter One 10

The Science behind Weight Loss 10

   Metabolism Demystified 11

   Nutritional Essential 13

   The Role of Exercise 17

Chapter Two 20

Building Healthy Habits 20

   Mindful Eating Technique 21

   Creating a Sustainable Workout Routine 25

   Sleep and Stress Management 28

Chapter Three 31

Navigating Challenges 31

   Overcoming Obstacles 31

   Managing Emotional Eating 33

   Dealing with Social Pressures 37

Chapter Four 40

Maintaining Success 40

   Maintenance Techniques..40

   Milestones to Remember...43

   Developing a Healthy Lifestyle for Life 46

Conclusion 49

Finding Your Way to a Healthier You 49

Introduction

Understanding the Weight Loss Journey

Embarking on a weight loss journey is a deeply personal and transforming process. It involves a range of physical, mental, and emotional changes that can have a tremendous impact on one's entire well-being. While losing weight may seem simple on the surface, the process is typically loaded with difficulties and challenges that demand determination, endurance, and a deep understanding of oneself.

One of the most critical components of understanding the weight reduction process is recognizing that it is not a fast fix or a temporary answer. Sustainable weight loss takes time, patience, and a long-term commitment to good practices. It demands a shift in thinking from wanting immediate results to embracing a healthier lifestyle that involves a nutritious diet and regular physical activity. By recognizing that weight loss is a gradual process, individuals can set realistic objectives and avoid the dangers of crash diets or drastic measures that are often unsustainable.

Another crucial facet of comprehending the weight reduction journey is realizing the value of self-reflection and self-acceptance. Many people embark on a weight loss journey because they wish to modify their looks or comply with societal standards. However, it is vital to remember that actual transformation goes beyond physical appearance. It involves loving oneself, establishing a positive body image, and fostering a balanced relationship with food and exercise. By fostering self-acceptance and practicing self-love, individuals can traverse the weight reduction process with a better sense of empowerment and confidence.

Understanding the weight reduction journey also entails comprehending the significance of mentality and motivation. Many people have experienced the frustration of starting a weight loss program with tremendous enthusiasm, only to lose motivation and relapse into old habits. Developing a strong mental framework and incentive system is vital for keeping on track. This includes defining clear and achievable goals, providing a supportive environment, and promoting a mindset that focuses on progress rather than perfection. By maintaining a good mindset and finding important incentives, individuals can stay motivated, overcome setbacks, and stay devoted to their weight reduction quest.

Furthermore, understanding the weight reduction process demands realizing the value of a comprehensive approach to health. It goes beyond just dropping pounds and involves entire well-being. This includes treating underlying problems like as stress, emotional eating, sleep patterns, and lifestyle choices. Seeking support from specialists such as dieticians, trainers, and therapists can provide vital direction and skills for individuals to handle these problems efficiently. By addressing the core reasons for weight gain and adding holistic practices into their daily routines, individuals can experience not only weight loss but also increased overall health.

Setting Realistic Goals

Setting realistic and achievable goals is a cornerstone of every successful weight reduction program. The challenge lies in establishing a balance between ambition and realism. Unrealistic goals can lead to dissatisfaction and burnout while setting the bar too low could not give the required challenge for progress.

When defining your weight loss goals, consider your starting point and your end objective. Break down your main goal into smaller, more doable benchmarks. For example, if your target is to lose 50 pounds, create intermediate goals of 5 or 10 pounds at a time. This not only makes the process more palatable but also helps you to enjoy tiny triumphs along the road.

Moreover, it's vital to make your goals explicit and measurable. Instead of a general objective like "I want to be healthier," consider specifying, "I will incorporate at least 30 minutes of moderate exercise into my routine five days a week." This precision helps you to track your progress and change your strategy if needed.

Consider the time frame for your goals as well. While it's tempting to want immediate results, sustainable weight loss frequently occurs gradually. Aim for a pace that allows your body to adjust and helps you develop permanent habits. Remember, it's not just about hitting a number on the scale but adopting a better lifestyle that you can maintain in the long run.

Lastly, be gentle to yourself. Understand that failures are a natural part of any journey, and flexibility in altering your goals may be empowering. Setting realistic goals is not about restricting your potential but rather ensuring that your aims correspond with what is feasible and maintained, encouraging a positive and successful weight reduction experience.

Chapter One

The Science behind Weight Loss

In this chapter, we dive into the deep science that governs the process of reducing excess weight. Understanding the physiological principles at play empowers you to make informed decisions, turning your weight loss journey into a science-backed pursuit.

Metabolism Demystified

Metabolism, sometimes termed the body's internal engine, is a complicated and dynamic process that directs the consumption of energy. At its core is the Basal Metabolic Rate (BMR), representing the calories your body needs at rest to maintain basic activities such as breathing and circulation. Understanding your BMR is vital as it establishes the framework for designing a successful weight loss strategy.

Factors regulating metabolism are various, and age plays a crucial impact. As we age, our metabolism begins to slow down, mostly due to a reduction in muscle mass. This highlights the need to include strength training activities into your routine, as growing and maintaining muscle can rev up your metabolic engine.

The Thermic Effect of Food (TEF) is another component of metabolism, representing the energy expended during the digestion and absorption of nutrients. Different macronutrients have varied TEF percentages, with proteins requiring more energy to digest compared to fats and carbs. Optimizing your diet to contain a balanced mix of these macronutrients can lead to a more efficient metabolism.

Contrary to prevalent notions, metabolism isn't only determined by heredity; lifestyle choices also play a key role. Regular physical activity, especially high-intensity interval training (HIIT), can boost your metabolism not only during the exercise itself but also in the post-exercise recovery period, known as excess post-exercise oxygen consumption (EPOC).

In essence, metabolism is a dynamic and complicated process driven by elements within and outside our control. By demystifying these factors, you obtain significant insights into how your body consumes energy, allowing you to make informed choices that can favorably impact your weight reduction journey.

Nutritional Essential

Nutritional requirements play a significant role in weight loss journeys as they give the necessary nutrients and fuel while promoting a healthy metabolism. One of the basic nutritional aspects necessary for weight loss is a balanced diet that contains all the major food groups. This involves consuming sufficient amounts of lean proteins, entire grains, fruits, vegetables, and healthy fats. Incorporating these foods into a weight loss strategy guarantees that the body receives critical vitamins, minerals, and antioxidants necessary for overall well-being.

Proper hydration is another dietary necessity in the context of weight loss. Drinking a proper amount of water throughout the day helps suppress appetite, improves digestion, and aids in the removal of waste and toxins from the body. In addition to water, introducing herbal teas, infused water, or low-calorie beverages can add variety while promoting hydration. Staying hydrated is not only advantageous for weight loss but also plays a critical role in maintaining energy levels and fostering normal body functions.

Adequate protein intake is crucial for weight loss due to its capacity to promote satiety, boost metabolism, and aid in muscle recovery and growth. Including lean sources of protein, such as poultry, fish, tofu, lentils, and Greek yogurt, can help individuals feel satiated for longer, minimizing the likelihood of overeating or snacking on harmful foods. Protein also plays a critical function in sustaining lean muscle mass during weight loss, ensuring that the majority of weight loss comes from fat rather than muscle. It is important to distribute protein consumption evenly throughout the day to maximize its advantages and boost weight loss attempt

Choosing the proper forms of carbs is vital in a weight loss quest. Complex carbs, such as whole grains, legumes, and vegetables, give a constant supply of energy and minimize blood sugar spikes and crashes. These carbs are rich in fiber, which aids in digestion, promotes feelings of fullness, and helps manage blood sugar levels. On the other hand, refined carbs, such as white bread, sugary snacks, and processed foods, should be minimized as they can lead to weight gain and impair weight loss success.

Healthy fats are sometimes misinterpreted in weight loss strategies. While it may seem contradictory, consuming the appropriate types of fats can aid in weight loss. Unsaturated fats, found in foods like avocados, almonds, seeds, and olive oil, are great for heart health and help increase feelings of fullness. They also play a role in nutritional absorption, as several vitamins are fat-soluble. However, it's crucial to consume fats in moderation, as they are high in calories. It's encouraged to focus on introducing healthy fats into meals and snacks instead of consuming them in excess.

In addition to these dietary necessities, portion control also plays a significant part in weight loss. Even if one includes all the necessary nutrients in their meals, ingesting excessive portions can lead to a calorie surplus and inhibit weight loss progress. It's crucial to be conscious of portion sizes and respond to the body's hunger cues. Incorporating practices like using smaller plates, monitoring amounts, and practicing mindful eating can help individuals maintain an optimal calorie intake for weight loss while still satisfying their nutritional needs.

In conclusion, a good diet is vital for weight loss since it provides the body with the necessary nutrients, boosts metabolism, and aids in maintaining energy levels. A balanced diet that includes lean proteins, complex carbohydrates, healthy fats, and hydration is vital. In addition, portion control and implementing mindful eating can further promote weight loss goals. By focusing on these nutritional necessities, individuals can boost their weight loss journeys and obtain sustained outcomes.

The Role of Exercise

Exercise is a dynamic catalyst in the weight loss path, reaching beyond simply calorie burning to modify your body composition and increase general well-being. Understanding the varied facets of exercise helps you to adapt your exercises for optimal impact.

Cardiovascular exercises, such as jogging, swimming, and cycling, boost your heart rate, promoting calorie expenditure and enhancing cardiovascular health. These workouts not only aid in weight loss but also boost endurance and stamina. Engaging in frequent cardio exercises boosts your metabolism, creating a more efficient calorie-burning process.

Strength training, frequently disregarded in typical weight loss approaches, is a tremendous tool for changing your body. Building lean muscle mass through sports like weightlifting not only boosts your metabolic rate but also creates a toned and sculpted appearance. Additionally, muscular tissue continues to burn calories even at rest, helping to maintain weight management.

Flexibility and balance exercises, implemented through practices like yoga and Pilates, offer overall advantages. They promote joint mobility, minimize the chance of accidents, and boost general body awareness. Integrating these exercises into your regimen provides a well-rounded approach to fitness and aids in recovery from more rigorous workouts.

High-intensity interval Training (HIIT) stands out as an efficient and time-effective training approach. Alternating between short bursts of intense activity and intervals of rest not only burns calories during the workout but also causes an afterburn effect known as excess post-exercise oxygen consumption (EPOC). This sustained calorie burn post-exercise adds to weight loss over time.

In essence, the importance of exercise in weight loss extends far beyond the chase of a number on the scale. It involves cardiovascular health, muscular strength, flexibility, and overall well-being. By embracing a diversified and balanced workout program, you not only optimize your weight loss efforts but also create a sustainable and pleasant commitment to fitness.

Chapter Two

Building Healthy Habits

Creating lasting change in your lifestyle is a vital part of a successful weight loss journey. Building healthy habits goes beyond quick cures, concentrating on cultivating behaviors that lead to long-term well-being. In this chapter, we cover fundamental tactics for building and keeping habits that support your health and weight loss goals.

Mindful Eating Technique

In today's fast-paced world, many individuals battle with weight control due to hectic schedules and bad eating habits. However, a practice known as mindful eating has attracted attention for its potential to aid in weight loss.

Mindful eating approaches involve being fully present and aware of the eating experience and developing a healthier connection with food. Let's investigate some effective mindful eating practices that can contribute to successful weight loss.

1. Eat with intention: Before each meal, set an intention to eat with purpose and mindfulness. This simple step helps shift the focus from thoughtless eating to consciously nourishing the body. Be conscious of your hunger cues and eat when you feel genuinely hungry.

2. Be present with your food: Engage all your senses while eating. Take a moment to appreciate the appearance, aroma, and texture of your meal. Chew carefully and relish each bite to enhance the eating experience. This exercise allows you to detect when you are full, preventing overeating.

3. Listen to your body: Pay attention to your body's indications of hunger and fullness. Eat until you are full, not until you are stuffed. Avoid distractions while eating, such as devices or multitasking, as these might isolate you from your body's natural signals.

4. Engage in mindful food choices: When making meal choices, exercise attentive awareness of what your body needs and craves. Consider the nutritional value and how different foods make you feel. Opt for whole, unadulterated foods that fuel your body rather than selecting empty calories.

5. Practice portion control: Mindful eating involves becoming aware of food sizes and serving yourself correctly. Use smaller dishes and bowls to help reduce portion sizes. Eat gently and take breaks during your meal to evaluate if you are still hungry or satisfied.

6. Cultivate thankfulness: Take a moment to express gratitude for the food you are about to eat. Mindful eating is about appreciating and being appreciative of the nourishment your food offers. This practice creates a positive view of food and encourages thoughtful choices.

7. Manage emotional eating: Emotional eating is a major challenge when it comes to losing weight. Mindfulness can assist in detecting emotional triggers that contribute to mindless eating. Instead of turning to food for comfort or distraction, consider finding alternate ways to handle your feelings, including practicing deep breathing, journaling, or indulging in a beloved hobby.

8. Slow down and savor meals: In our hectic lives, meals are often rushed or consumed on the go. Engaging in mindful eating involves taking the time to slow down and fully relish each meal. Take small nibbles, chew carefully, and thoroughly absorb the flavors and sensations of your food. This not only helps you enjoy your food more but also allows your brain to notice when you're satisfied, preventing overeating.

9. Practice attentive snacking: Snacking often contributes to weight gain, especially when it's driven by thoughtless eating. Instead, employ mindful snacking practices to make healthier choices. Before grabbing a snack, ask yourself if you're hungry or if you're eating out of boredom or stress. Choose nutritious selections like fruits, veggies, or a handful of nuts, and savor them carefully.

10. Reflect on your eating experience: After each meal, take a moment to reflect on your experience. How did the food make you feel? Were you satisfied? Did you enjoy the flavors? This reflection helps improve self-awareness and prompts adjustments for future meals, leading to a more mindful and well-balanced approach to eating.

Recall that developing the ability of mindful eating takes time. Start by adopting one or two techniques and gradually build upon them. By being present and conscious of your eating patterns, you may build a healthier relationship with food and assist your weight loss journey.

Creating a Sustainable Workout Routine

Establishing an exercise regimen that endures the test of time is vital for achieving and sustaining your weight loss objectives. Sustainability is the key, and that entails selecting things that you enjoy, setting reasonable objectives, and introducing variation into your routines.

Firstly, identify activities that resonate with you. Whether it's brisk walking, jogging, cycling, dancing, or weightlifting, picking exercises that correspond with your interest means that you're more likely to persist with them over the long term. Enjoying your workouts changes fitness from a chore to a joyful and meaningful component of your routine.

Setting realistic goals is crucial for sustainability. While aspiration is wonderful, it's vital to identify your present fitness level and steadily advance. Establish achievable milestones that keep you engaged without risking fatigue or harm. Celebrating these tiny achievements leads to a happy and reinforcing fitness experience.

Variety is the spice of life, and it applies to your training routine as well. Incorporate several sorts of exercises to keep things interesting and minimize monotony. Cross-training not only targets numerous muscle groups but also minimizes the chance of overuse problems. Experiment with different fitness classes, outdoor activities, or training types to discover what keeps you focused and excited.

Consistency is the backbone of a sustainable training plan. Treat your workout sessions as non-negotiable appointments, prioritizing them in your agenda. Creating a routine entails setting a regular workout time, whether it's in the morning, during lunch, or in the evening. Consistency strengthens the habit, making exercise a vital part of your everyday life.

Remember, the objective is not just to reduce weight but to build a lifelong relationship with fitness. By picking fun activities, setting reasonable goals, introducing diversity, and keeping consistent, you create a fitness routine that becomes a sustainable and pleasurable part of your everyday. This strategy ensures that exercise is not simply a means to an end but a fulfilling and enduring journey.

Sleep and Stress Management

Sleep is a critical component of healthy weight loss and stress management. Numerous studies have demonstrated a substantial correlation between poor sleep and weight growth. When individuals do not get enough sleep, their hormone levels become imbalanced, resulting in increased hunger and cravings for high-calorie, unhealthy meals. This leads to overconsumption and difficulty in keeping a healthy diet. In addition, lack of sleep can severely affect energy levels and motivation to engage in physical activity, producing a drop in calorie expenditure. Therefore, prioritizing sleep is vital for weight loss by helping to regulate hunger and boosting general well-being.

Stress management plays a crucial part in weight loss as it affects both physical and psychological variables. Chronic stress can lead to the formation of abdominal fat, also known as visceral fat, which is related to an increased risk of different health concerns such as heart disease and type 2 diabetes. This is due to the release of stress hormones such as cortisol, which increases the storage of fat, particularly in the abdominal area. Moreover, stress can prompt emotional eating as a coping technique, frequently involving the consumption of unhealthy, calorie-dense foods to momentarily reduce tension and bring comfort. Developing good stress management skills, such as exercise, mindfulness practices, and relaxation techniques, can help in reducing stress levels and minimizing weight gain connected with stress.

Integrating adequate sleep and stress management measures into a weight reduction program can considerably boost its success. Adequate sleep allows the body to recover and repair itself, optimizing metabolism and energy levels for optimal weight loss results. Moreover, quality sleep helps regulate the synthesis of hormones that affect hunger and satiety, reducing the probability of overeating. In terms of stress management, adopting appropriate coping methods helps minimize emotional eating and develop a positive mentality, which is vital for sustaining long-term weight loss objectives. By prioritizing sleep and managing stress properly, individuals can create a conducive atmosphere for weight loss and overall well-being.

Implementing sleep and stress management strategies demands a commitment to healthy lifestyle practices. Establishing a consistent sleep schedule, regulating sleep surroundings, and practicing relaxation techniques before bed can increase the quality of sleep. Additionally, engaging in regular physical activity not only benefits stress management but also improves sleep quality. Incorporating stress-reducing activities such as yoga, deep breathing exercises, and meditation can help individuals better manage stress and minimize the chance of stress-induced weight gain. Recognizing the importance of sleep and stress management as vital aspects of a weight reduction journey can pave the path to long-lasting success and improved overall health. It is crucial to emphasize self-care and make these activities a priority to optimize weight loss efforts and build a balanced and healthy lifestyle.

Chapter Three

Navigating Challenges

Starting a weight loss journey is a noble goal, but it is not without its difficulties. In this chapter, we look at frequent roadblocks and offer solutions to help you stay resilient and devoted to your goals.

Overcoming Obstacles

Obstacles are a normal component of the weight loss process, indicating a temporary halt in progress. Understanding and accepting this phenomenon is critical to properly navigating it. When you reach a plateau, avoid the desire to give up and instead see it as an opportunity for reconsideration and refining.

Reevaluating your food and exercise routine is a great method for breaking through plateaus. Examine your calorie intake to ensure it corresponds to your current weight and activity level. Adjusting your caloric intake, whether through small decreases or the addition of nutrient-dense foods, might rekindle your body's response to weight loss efforts.

Another important factor in breaking over plateaus is variety. Introduce new activities or make changes to your current workout regimen to target different muscle groups. This not only keeps you from becoming bored, but it also stimulates your body in ways that may help you break through the plateau. Consider adding interval training, experimenting with new types of cardio, or raising the intensity of your strength sessions.

During plateaus, consistency is quite important. Maintain your healthy practices and have faith in the process. Remember that weight swings are normal, and long-term success frequently requires periods of slower development. Celebrate non-scale achievements, such as increased energy, improved fitness, or improved mood, to encourage your commitment beyond the scale numbers.

By handling plateaus with patience, adaptability, and a positive outlook, you can turn them from roadblocks to stepping stones on your weight reduction path. Accept the chance for self-reflection and correction, understanding that perseverance and adaptation are the keys to breaking through plateaus and reaching your ultimate goals.

Managing Emotional Eating

Dealing with emotional eating is a typical difficulty for many people on their weight reduction journey. Emotional eating is the practice of turning to food as a coping mechanism for unpleasant feelings including stress, sadness, boredom, or even happiness.

It can be a significant impediment to weight loss objectives because it frequently leads to overeating and the consumption of bad, calorie-dense meals.

It is critical to recognize the triggers and underlying feelings that contribute to emotional eating to properly deal with it and assist in weight loss attempts. Recognizing the behaviors and conditions that trigger emotional eating episodes requires self-awareness. Keeping a food journal can help individuals track their eating habits and identify emotional triggers, allowing them to have a better understanding of their connection with food.

Another important part of regulating emotional eating is the development of alternate coping skills. Finding better outlets for emotions, such as exercising, reading, meditating, or engaging in hobbies, might be beneficial instead of turning to food. These activities serve to divert attention away from food and provide healthy outlets for stress or other emotions.

Having a strong support network may also be helpful in overcoming emotional eating. During difficult times, friends, family, and even support groups can provide important encouragement, empathy, and understanding. Engaging with others who are on the same weight reduction path as you help foster a feeling of community, making it easier to keep motivated and accountable.

Mindful eating is another helpful strategy for combating emotional eating. Mindful eating entails paying complete attention to the eating experience - savoring each bite, chewing deeply, and being mindful of physical hunger and fullness signs. Individuals can distinguish between actual physical hunger and emotional hunger by focusing on the current moment and making healthier decisions as a result.

In addition to these measures, it is critical to develop a healthy eating plan that includes a range of whole foods.

Including enough protein, fiber, and healthy fats in each meal can help people feel fuller for longer and minimize cravings, which can contribute to emotional eating. Prioritizing sufficient water is particularly important, as dehydration can sometimes be misinterpreted as hunger, leading to unnecessary snacking.

Finally, getting professional assistance, such as counseling or therapy, can help to address the underlying emotional issues that contribute to emotional eating. A competent therapist can assist people in developing healthier coping methods, managing stress, and developing a positive relationship with food.

Managing emotional eating in the context of weight loss requires patience, self-compassion, and willingness to address underlying emotional issues. Individuals can effectively manage emotional eating and support their weight loss goals by identifying triggers, creating alternative coping methods, developing a support system, practicing mindful eating, following a balanced eating plan, and seeking professional treatment. It may not be an easy road, but it is possible to overcome emotional eating and live a healthier, happier life with dedication and determination.

Dealing with Social Pressures

Navigating social influences is a major obstacle in the weight reduction path, particularly in a world where social gatherings frequently focus on food. Maintaining your commitment to a better lifestyle in the face of social expectations requires assertiveness and strategic planning.

Communicating your intentions to friends and family can be an effective method for dealing with social constraints. Share your aims and the significance of your health journey to help others comprehend your dedication. This open conversation can build support and reduce external pressures to engage in unhealthy eating behaviors at social gatherings.

When confronted with social events involving food, planning ahead of time is a proactive tactic. Eat a nutritious lunch before going to an event to satisfy hunger and limit the possibility of overindulging. Bring healthy snacks or foods to share, and make sure some selections correspond with your dietary objectives. This not only helps you stay on track, but it also introduces others to healthy options.

It is critical to be aggressive in your choices. Politely decline offers of high-calorie foods or beverages that do not correspond to your aims. Remember that it is perfectly OK to prioritize your health and well-being. Developing the ability to say "no" when necessary allows you to make decisions that support your long-term goals while avoiding external constraints.

Find like-minded people or support groups with comparable health goals. Having a network of people with similar goals provides support and understanding.

Surrounding yourself with people who support your decisions can help reduce the influence of societal pressures and strengthen your commitment to a healthier lifestyle.

Handling social pressures entails a combination of communication, strategic planning, assertiveness, and the formation of a supportive network. By proactively addressing these barriers, you empower yourself to stick to your weight loss objectives while still engaging in social activities and living a healthy and meaningful life.

Chapter Four

Maintaining Success

Reaching your weight loss objectives is a huge accomplishment, but the road does not stop there. Sustaining success entails shifting from specialized weight loss tactics to a lifestyle that promotes long-term well-being. In this chapter, we will look at the fundamental elements of retaining your accomplishments and embracing a better, more balanced lifestyle.

Maintenance Techniques

Transitioning from active weight reduction to maintenance is a critical stage that necessitates a methodical and long-term approach. Maintenance techniques go beyond the specific tactics used during weight loss to create a lifestyle that promotes long-term well-being.

Consistent Healthy Habits: Maintaining the healthy habits that contributed to your weight reduction achievement is the foundation of maintenance. Maintain a healthy, nutrient-dense diet, regular physical activity, and appropriate sleep. Maintaining consistency in these behaviors guarantees that the improvement you've made becomes a part of your everyday routine.

Thoughtful Eating: Developing a thoughtful attitude to eating is essential for long-term success. Pay attention to hunger and fullness cues, taste the flavors of your meals, and choose portion amounts with care. Mindful eating promotes not only weight maintenance but also a pleasant relationship with food.

Regular Exercise schedule: Make physical activity a regular part of your schedule. Find activities that you enjoy to make exercise a long-term and pleasurable part of your life. Maintaining a regular exercise regimen, whether it's going for a walk, taking fitness classes, or participating in sports, is critical for overall health and weight management.

Periodic Assessments: Evaluate your behaviors and progress regularly. Examine your weight, exercise levels, and overall health regularly. If you find any deviations, take the initiative to address them. Change your habits or seek help to keep minor setbacks from becoming major issues.

Balanced diet: Move away from rigid calorie counting and toward a more balanced and intuitive approach to diet. Continue to eat full, nutrient-dense foods while allowing for occasional indulgences. The idea is to develop a long-term and joyful relationship with food that is not restrictive.

Stay Hydrated: Adequate hydration is frequently forgotten, but it is an essential component of living a healthy lifestyle. Drink plenty of water throughout the day, as hydration affects several biological functions, including metabolism and appetite regulation.

In essence, maintenance tactics entail incorporating the healthy behaviors you've formed during your weight reduction journey into the fabric of your daily life. You establish the framework for a sustainable and enjoyable lifestyle that promotes your long-term well-being by embracing consistency, mindfulness, regular evaluations, a balanced approach to diet, and staying hydrated.

Milestones to Remember

Celebrating weight reduction achievements is more than simply an acknowledgment; it's a strong tool for reinforcing positive behavior and retaining motivation. Milestones, whether large or small, serve as indicators of progress, reminding you of your accomplishments along the way.

Recognizing and celebrating weight-related milestones, such as reaching a certain weight or losing a certain percentage of body fat, provides a sense of accomplishment. Consider making a visual representation of your accomplishments, such as a progress chart or a before-and-after photo comparison, to help you see and appreciate the changes more clearly.

Non-scale victories are equally important in marking anniversaries. Improvements in fitness, energy, sleep quality, and mood are examples of such benefits. Recognize these accomplishments because they reflect the overall impact of your lifestyle changes, which contribute to a healthier and happier you.

To make the celebration more tangible, create a system of rewards for reaching milestones. Treat yourself to something special, such as a spa day, new clothing, or your favorite healthy meal. These incentives foster positive associations with your accomplishments, making the journey more enjoyable and reinforcing your dedication.

Share your achievements with a support system, whether it's family, friends, or an online community. Sharing your accomplishments not only increases your joy but also strengthens your social network by providing encouragement and positive reinforcement. Celebrating milestones as a group fosters a sense of belonging and accomplishment.

In essence, celebrating milestones is an essential practice on the road to long-term success. By recognizing and rewarding your accomplishments, you create a positive feedback loop that fuels motivation, reinforces positive behavior, and sets the stage for continued weight loss progress.

A successful weight loss journey is more than just a number on the scale; it is a transformation into a lifestyle that prioritizes long-term well-being. Cultivating a lifelong healthy lifestyle involves a shift in mindset from short-term goals to sustained, holistic health.

Embrace the concept of health as a journey rather than a destination. Rather than viewing your weight loss journey as a temporary effort, adopt a mindset that recognizes the ongoing nature of self-improvement and well-being. This shift ensures that healthy habits become an integral part of your identity and daily routine.

Continuous education is a cornerstone of cultivating a lifelong healthy lifestyle. Stay informed about nutrition, exercise, and mental well-being. As the field of health evolves, being knowledgeable empowers you to make informed decisions that align with the latest research and best practices, ensuring your lifestyle remains current and effective.

Incorporate variety into your routines to keep them engaging and sustainable. Experiment with different types of exercise, try new recipes and explore various wellness practices. Variety not only prevents monotony but also allows you to discover what resonates most with you, enhancing the enjoyment and longevity of your healthy lifestyle.

Make self-care a top priority in your daily routine. Whether it's taking time for relaxation, pursuing hobbies, or engaging in activities that bring you joy, self-care is vital for mental and emotional well-being. A balanced lifestyle that nurtures your mind, body, and spirit contributes to sustained health and happiness.

Be adaptable and resilient in the face of challenges. Life is dynamic, and circumstances may change. A flexible approach allows you to adjust your strategies, goals, and routines to align with evolving priorities, ensuring that your healthy lifestyle remains realistic and attainable.

In essence, cultivating a lifelong healthy lifestyle is a commitment to continual growth, self-care, and adaptability. By embracing health as an ongoing journey, staying informed, incorporating variety, prioritizing self-care, and maintaining flexibility, you lay the foundation for a lifestyle that not only sustains your weight loss achievements but also fosters enduring well-being.

Conclusion

Finding Your Way to a Healthier You

As we get to the end of our journey together, it's important to take stock of the significant changes that have occurred in addition to the weight loss. Losing weight is more than just a number; it's a deep self-examination, a dedication to health, and an example of resiliency.

We've examined the intricacies of diet and exercise, descended into the science of weight loss, and tackled the psychological and social aspects of the process in these pages. We've overcome obstacles, rejoiced in successes, and established the foundation for long-term success. However, this is only the beginning of a lifelong commitment to health; it is not the end.

Keep in mind that the decisions you make every day to take care of your body and mind determine your value rather than the number on the scale. A healthy lifestyle is a dynamic, ever-changing endeavor that values flexibility, self-awareness, and ongoing development.

Carry with you the wisdom acquired, the lessons discovered, and the fortitude developed by adversity as you forward. Celebrate the person you've become along the way as well as the accomplishments you've made. Your route to well-being is a personal story that develops with every deliberate decision and constructive deed; your journey is distinct.

Accept that maintaining your health is a comprehensive process that requires ongoing learning, self-care, and flexibility. This book is a guide, a traveling partner on your continuous journey to a better, happier version of yourself, not the end.

I hope you make healthy decisions every day, overcome obstacles with fortitude, and joyfully enjoy your accomplishments. Cheers to the power of transformation that resides within you and the ongoing development of your well-being. A healthier you is the result of a journey, not a destination, and it is on this journey that life begins to reveal itself.

I would be very grateful if you could give this book a review and rating on Amazon. Your criticism enables me to write better and connect with more readers like you. I appreciate your help.